Reine BAHAYA MULUZINYERE

Dental caries and associated factors:

Reine BAHAYA MULUZINYERE

Dental caries and associated factors:

study of children aged 5-6, 12 and 15 from North and South Kivu in the Democratic Republic of Congo

ScienciaScripts

Imprint
Any brand names and product names mentioned in this book are subject to trademark, brand or patent protection and are trademarks or registered trademarks of their respective holders. The use of brand names, product names, common names, trade names, product descriptions etc. even without a particular marking in this work is in no way to be construed to mean that such names may be regarded as unrestricted in respect of trademark and brand protection legislation and could thus be used by anyone.

Cover image: www.ingimage.com

This book is a translation from the original published under ISBN 978-620-6-69029-0.

Publisher:
Sciencia Scripts
is a trademark of
Dodo Books Indian Ocean Ltd. and OmniScriptum S.R.L publishing group

120 High Road, East Finchley, London, N2 9ED, United Kingdom
Str. Armeneasca 28/1, office 1, Chisinau MD-2012, Republic of Moldova, Europe
Printed at: see last page
ISBN: 978-620-8-13960-5

I dedicate this book

My Friend and Husband Professor Alumeti Munyali Désiré

My children Christian Anthonya Alumeti, Christelle Ambika Alumeti, and Christophe Mukengere Alumeti.

This book is the fruit of your love for Me.

My dear parents, Papa Elias Bahaya and Maman Marie-Rose M'Katembera

To Professor Malick Faye

To the Alimeti and BAHAYA families

To the DIOP and DIA families

To the Denis Mukwege Family

To all our family friends

To the children of North and South Kivu

May this book breathe new life into the problems of oral health in North and South Kivu in the Democratic Republic of Congo.

To the Medical Staff at Panzi Hospital and the entire team at the Evangelical University in Africa, may this book be a source of inspiration for developing public health programs in our environment.

(Queen Muluzinyere BAHAYA)

ACKNOWLEDGEMENTS

The authors would like to thank the Fondation Panzi / RDC and the Université Evangélique en Afrique for their financial support. They would also like to thank the heads of various hospitals and the entire team of the Pediatric Odontology Department at Cheikh Anta Diop University for their support and participation in the study.

Our most heartfelt thanks, for their invaluable contributions, to: -Pr Denis M. Mukwege: Chairman of the Board of Directors of the Panzi Foundation / DR-Congo; Mail:dm-cabinet@ hopitaldepanzi.org

• Professor Malick Faye: Head of the Pediatric Odontology Department at Cheikh Anta Diop University (UCAD); Mail: malick.faye@ucad.edu.sn

• Pr Ngongo Kilongo Fatuma, Rector of the Evangelical University in Africa; Mail: mangokifa@gmail .com

• Pr Mushagalusa Nachigera Gustave, Honorary Rector of the Université Evangélique en Afrique; Mail: nachigera@uea.ac.cd

• Pr Alumeti Munyali: Dean of the Faculty of Medicine at the Université Evangélique en Afrique(UEA); Mail: dr.alumetimunyali@gmail.com

• Pr Katcho Karhume: Honorary Dean of the Faculty of Agricultural and Environmental Sciences at the Evangelical University in Africa; Mail: kkatcho@yahoo.com

• Pr Charles Pilipili: Dean of Odontostomatology, Université des Montagnes-Bangangte - Cameroon; Mail: charles.pilipili@icloud.com

-Dr Soukeye Ndoye: Assistant Professor in the Department of Pediatric Odontology at Cheikh Anta Diop University (UCAD); Mail: souksbill@hotmail.com

- Dr Grace M. Kadimanche: Dental surgeon Hôpital Malkia wa Amani- Bukavu RDC; Mail: kadimanchemukebayi@gmail .com

Many thanks to Dr. Agbor Ashu Michael, Ir Yannick Mugumaarhahama and Pr. Bagalwa Mashimango, for their support.

TABLE OF CONTENTS

INTRODUCTION 5

CHAPTER I: GENERAL INFORMATION ON DENTAL CARIES 7

CHAPTER II: PRESENTATION OF THE STUDY FRAMEWORK: NORTH AND SOUTH KIVU/RD CONGO 11

CHAPTER III: DENTAL CARIES AND ASSOCIATED FACTORS: A STUDY OF CHILDREN IN NORTH AND SOUTH KIVU IN THE DEMOCRATIC REPUBLIC OF CONGO 13

CONCLUSION AND RECOMMENDATION 37

REFERENCES 38

PUBLICATIONS 46

INTRODUCTION

Dental caries is a multifactorial disease caused by an alteration in the composition of the bacterial biofilm, leading to an imbalance between demineralization and remineralization processes **(1)**. It is the most common childhood disease, affecting 60-90% of school-age children, and is responsible for millions of lost school days every year **(2)**. It is strongly linked to the patient's dietary habits, sugar intake, salivary flow, salivary fluoride levels and dental preventive behaviours **(3,4)**. Poor populations are still largely affected **(5).** In developed countries, the prevalence of dental caries is declining due to the installation of community dental facilities and the introduction of prevention programs **(6),** whereas an unprecedented increase in prevalence is reported in developing countries due to the growing consumption of sugary foods, insufficient exposure to fluorides, poor tooth-brushing habits, and lack of adequate dental services **(6 , 7, 8)**. In contrast to other age groups, studies among young people remain rare and are mainly conducted in high-income countries **(10)**. Little information is available on the prevalence of dental caries in children in the Democratic Republic of Congo, and particularly in the provinces of North and South Kivu, and most data is not available on common search engines (**10 11**). The provinces of North and South Kivu are among the poorest in the country, with political instability and armed conflict complicating the daily survival of the inhabitants **(12,13).** Data from the health pyramids of the 2020 health zones showed that the population of these two provinces was 17881122 (**14,15**), while data from the National Oral Health Program on health infrastructures and resources showed that there were 22 structures providing oral health care and 18 dentists spread across the two regions, giving a ratio of 1:993,395 inhabitants, compared with the World Health Organization's ratio of 1:10,000 (**14 ,15**). In some parts of these provinces, access to quality healthcare is perceived by the population as a difficult objective to achieve, either because of low income, or the remoteness or even absence of health structures (**16,17**). There is a significant need for oral health care, which cannot be met due to a largely inadequate and unevenly distributed supply of care.

In this context, the prevalence, severity and factors associated with dental caries should be continuously assessed in these two regions using suitable detection indices; this will enable disease progression to be halted and controlled through remineralization of lesions before they progress to a cavity. In recent decades, a wide variety of new methods have been developed to measure caries in a population **(18 ,19).** These include the Caries Severity Index (CAD) recommended by the World Health Organization (WHO), and the new *International Caries Detection and Assessment System* (ICDAS) (**20,22**). This ICDAS index allows standardized collection of caries data in different situations, and enables better comparison between studies (**22,23**). ICDAS prides itself on providing crucial data to aid decision-making when implementing preventive and therapeutic programs. It is also widely used in dental education, clinical practice, research and epidemiology **(2, 20**).

The aim of this book is to present the results of two research projects on dental caries and associated factors in children in North and South Kivu.

In the first chapter, this work will deal with the general aspects of dental caries in children, covering the etiopathogenic mechanisms, the risk factors involved, the caries indices used to describe the state of health of a population, and the treatment of dental caries.

In the second chapter, we present the study setting, North and South Kivu in the Democratic Republic of Congo.

Before concluding, the third chapter looks at the methodology applied and the results obtained from two separate studies:

- —A study of the frequency of caries in children attending dental services in public and private hospitals in North and South Kivu;
- —A school-based epidemiological study to assess the prevalence and severity of dental caries in children aged 5-6, 12 and 15 in North and South Kivu, and to determine the factors associated with dental caries in children in these two regions.

CHAPTER I: GENERAL INFORMATION ON DENTAL CARIES

Children are frequently affected by pathologies such as dental caries, periodontal disease, trauma and other abnormalities. These pathologies can have more serious consequences due to the immaturity of the child's defense systems, his or her state of growth and the lesser mineralization of the teeth (**24**).

1. Definition

1.1. According to the WHO

Caries is defined as "a localized pathological process, of external origin, appearing after eruption, accompanied by softening of the hard tissues and evolving towards the formation of a cavity" (**25**).

1.2. According to the ORCA/IADR Cariology Research Group consensus

Dental caries is a dynamic, multifactorial, non-transmissible, diet-modulated, biofilm-mediated disease, resulting in net mineral loss from hard dental tissues. It is determined by biological, behavioral, psychosocial and environmental factors. As a result of this process, a carious lesion develops (**26**)

2. Epidemiology

Dental caries is the most widespread chronic disease in the world, and a major public health issue (**27, 28**). It is the most common disease of childhood, affecting 573 million children (**29,30**).

The global prevalence of untreated permanent tooth decay is over 40%, affecting 44% of the world's population in 2010, followed by tension headache (21%), migraine (15%), periodontitis (11%), diabetes (8%) and asthma (5%) (**30, 31**).

In DR-Congo, few studies have been carried out on the oral health status of children. According to the Programme Nationale de Santé Bucco-Dentaire(RDC) , data from a few provincial health facilities, NGOs working at community level, and end-of-cycle work by dental students (2011-2016) show a high rate of dental caries in the 0-10 age group, followed by the 11-19 age group (**32**).

Knowledge of the distribution of tooth decay enables us to identify the factors likely to modify its incidence (**33**). Once confirmed by analytical surveys, risk factors can be controlled through intervention epidemiology. Finally, dental caries can be prevented (primary prevention), treated (secondary prevention) or its complications managed (tertiary prevention) (**20**).

3. Etiopathogenesis of dental caries

As early as 1946, Keyes identified three main etiological factors in the development of the dynamic process of tooth decay: the host, microbial factors and diet, to which Newbrun, in 1978, added the time factor (**34**).

Today, dental caries is considered a multifactorial disease, showing the interrelation between biological and social factors (**35**). (figure 1).

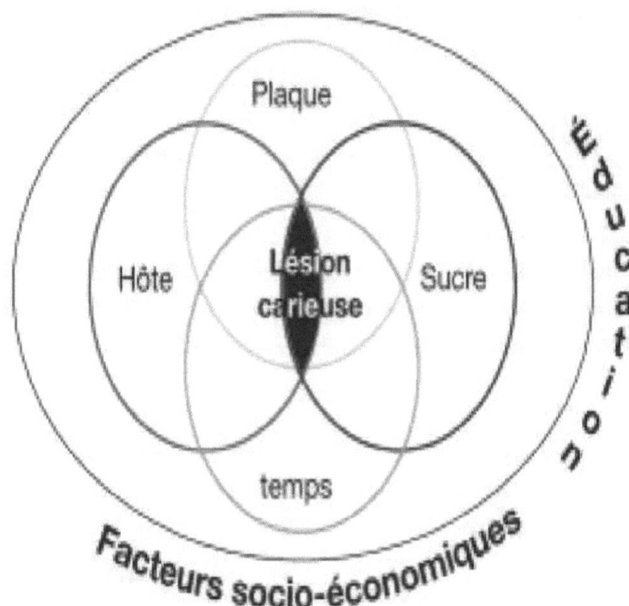

Figure 1: Keyes diagram modified by Newbrun and revised by Reisne and Douglas (175)

4. Risk factors for caries genesis

A large number of susceptibility factors have since been incriminated, making caries a multifactorial disease (figure 3).

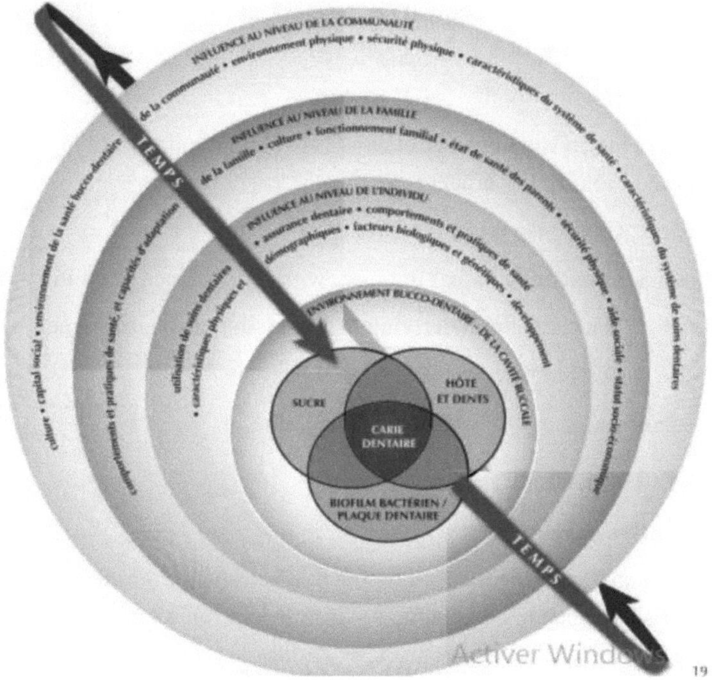

Figure 2: Tooth decay is a multifactorial disease: adapted from Fisher-Owens, 2007 (35)

5. Caries indicators

Indices are used to assess the oral health status of an individual or a population at a given point in time. In most cases, they are used in epidemiological studies published worldwide. These indices enable comparisons to be made over time or space, as well as highlighting the level of effectiveness of preventive measures or therapies applied (**36**). For the purposes of this book, we will apply the ICDAS index.

The ICDAS (*International Caries Detection Assessment System)* index is recommended by EGOHID (*European Global Oral Health Indicators Development*) because it improves the detection of suspected caries lesions not detectable with the conventional CAD method.

ICDAS has the advantage of providing crucial data for the choice of preventive and therapeutic programs **(20).**

ICDAS codes for detecting coronal carious lesions range from 0 to 6, depending on the severity of the lesion.

- Code 0: Healthy tooth
- Code1: First visual enamel change (visible only after prolonged drying or confined to pits and cracks)
- Code 2: Clear visual change of enamel
- Code 3: Localized enamel fracture (without evidence of dentinal damage)
- Code 4: Dark area in underlying dentin visible through enamel
- Code 5: Distinct cavity with exposed dentine
- Code 6: Large cavity with exposed dentine

6. Tooth decay therapy

6.1. Preventive care

Most clinical studies have focused on the evaluation of fluoride therapy, the use of pit and fissure sealants or plaque control. It is a function of individual caries risk (ICR) (**37**).

6.2. Curative Care

Lesions showing cavitation are the only ones suitable for restorative treatment. If the lesion is already developed, the new conservative approach - "minimal adhesive dentistry" - allows for micro-cavitation and controlled placement of adhesives and materials.

CHAPTER II: PRESENTATION OF THE STUDY FRAMEWORK: NORTH AND SOUTH KIVU/RD CONGO

1. Physical situation

The Provinces of North and South Kivu are the result of the division of ex-Kivu into three test provinces, namely Maniema, North and South Kivu, by Ordinance-Law no. 88- 031 of July 20 1988 (**38**) (figure 3).

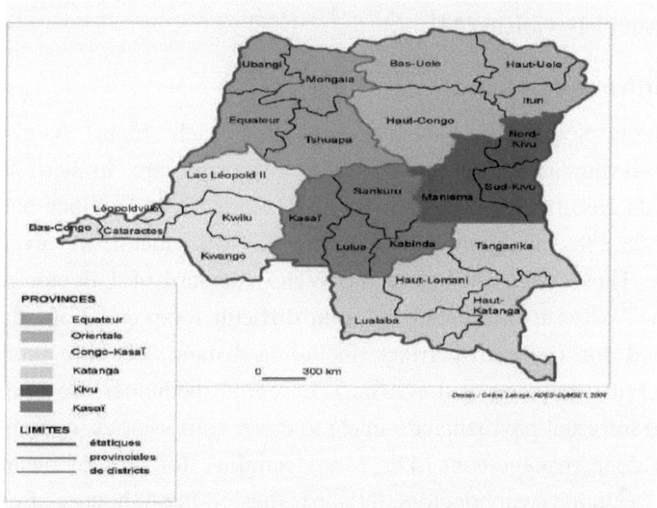

Figure 3: North and South Kivu before division (39)

Goma is the capital of North Kivu province. It comprises 6 territories: Beni, Lubero, Rutshuru, Walikale, Masisi and Nyiragongo. It covers an area of 59631km^2 and has an estimated population of 9,939,612, 64% of whom live in rural areas. Children under 5 account for 20% of the population, and 57% are under 18. Average household size is 6.0 (**40, 41**).

South Kivu province occupies 3% of the country's surface area, or 69130 km^2 . Its total population in 2020 was 7,941,510, 47% of whom lived in rural areas. The province has 22% of children under the age of 5, with 61% of the population under the age of 18, and an average household size of 5.9 (135). It has eight territories, including Fizi, Idjwi, Kabare, Walungu, Kalehe, Mwenga Shabunda and Uvira, and five towns, including Kamituga, Shabunda, Uvira, Baraka and Bukavu, the provincial capital (**42, 43**).

2. Living conditions

North and South Kivu are among the poorest provinces in the DRC. Their populations are very young, with half under the age of 18. The agricultural sector provides more than 7 out of every 10 jobs (**41**). For the past two decades, they have faced armed conflicts that have led to massive and recurrent population displacements, serious human rights violations and the collapse of basic social services. The presence of numerous active armed groups makes the security situation extremely violent (**44).**

3. Health organization

Both North and South Kivu have 34 health zones each **(45,46).** As elsewhere in the DRC, health structures are fragile, resources are limited and health professionals are often unqualified. In 2009, North Kivu province had 1 doctor for every 23,328 inhabitants, and South Kivu 1 doctor for every 27,699 inhabitants. These rates are below the WHO standard of 1 doctor per 10,000 inhabitants. Access to healthcare is often difficult for populations due to both financial and non-financial barriers (including distance between home and the point of service delivery, and conflict). Essential medicines are often in short supply, and informal payments are made to cover staff salaries, operational costs and health zone management (**47**). Many families, for lack of means, turn to traditional medicine (witchdoctors, fetishists, healers) or to houses of prayer (**40**).

4. Oral health situation (SBD)

The DRC's National Oral Health Program has a National or Central Coordination, which does not yet have a head office, and Provincial Coordinations.

North and South Kivu have 22 facilities providing oral health care **(32**). However, in the country's current context, the technical facilities available to these different services and/or practices are insufficient to fully carry out the tasks assigned to them.

Of the 716 dentists in the DRC in 2019, 9 were in North Kivu (a ratio of 1 dentist per 1,104,401 inhabitants, compared with the WHO standard of 1 per 10,000 inhabitants) and 9 in South Kivu (a ratio of 1 dentist per 882,390 inhabitants)(**32**).

There are also a small number of nurses who are trained in oral health by certain colleagues in their dental practices. (**32**)

CHAPTER III: DENTAL CARIES AND ASSOCIATED FACTORS: A STUDY OF CHILDREN IN NORTH AND SOUTH KIVU IN THE DEMOCRATIC REPUBLIC OF CONGO

Study №1: Frequency of dental caries in children: a study carried out in the dental services of North and South Kivu in the Democratic Republic of Congo.

1.1. INTRODUCTION

Dental caries has a high incidence and prevalence, and is one of the most widespread diseases in the world (**48**). Few studies have been carried out on the prevalence of dental caries among children in Kinshasa (**49**).

However, few studies have been carried out in North and South Kivu (**50**).

The aim of this study was to determine the prevalence of caries disease in children aged 5, 12 and 15 who consulted dental services in public and private hospitals in North and South Kivu from 2009 to 2019.

1.2. METHODOLOGY

This was a retrospective study of children aged 5, 12 and 15 who consulted dental services in North and South Kivu from 2009 to 2019. These different ages were selected according to WHO recommendations for oral surveys.

The WHO recommends the following ages and age ranges: 5 years for baby teeth, 12 years, 15 years, 35-44 years and 65-74 years for permanent teeth **(51).**

The presence of a dental surgeon and the existence of patient files or registers were the criteria used to select the facilities.

Geographical location, reputation and willingness to collaborate with researchers enabled us to select 13 public and private structures.

Authorization from the heads of the departments concerned was requested beforehand.

Thus, correctly completed registers or records of patients aged 5, 12 and 15 years were included in the study.

The data were collected from the registers using a pre-defined data sheet.

Information on age, sex, address, year of first consultation, reason for consultation and data on the clinical examination itself (diagnosis, number and type of decayed teeth) were obtained.

The data collected were entered into Microsoft Excel 2013, then analyzed using SPSS version 23 software. Quantitative variables were described by mean and standard deviation. Categorical variables (gender, origin, tooth type) were described by frequency and number. The Pearson chi-square test was used to compare proportions. Results were considered significant at the 5% uncertainty level ($p < 0.05$).

1.3. RESULTS

The study involved 3,222 children, with 988 (30.7%) in North Kivu and 2,234 (69.3%) in South Kivu. The sex ratio was 0.82, i.e. 1453 (45.1%) boys to 1769 (54.9%) girls. The sample was mainly made up of children aged 5 (54.7%), 94.85% of whom lived in urban areas (Table I).

Table I: General characteristics of the sample

Features	North Kivu N (%)	South Kivu N (%)	Total N (%)
Number of consultations	998 (30,7)	2234 (69,3)	3222 (100)
Gender			
Female	550 (17,07)	1219 (37,83)	1769 (54,92)
Male	438 (13,6)	1014 (31,47)	1453 (45,08)
Age (years)			
Five	476 (14,77)	1288 (39,97)	1764 (54,75)
Twelve	310 (9,62)	434 (13,46)	744 (23,09)
Fifteen	202 (6,26)	512 (15,58)	714 (22,16)
Provenance			
Urban	909 (92,00)	2118 (94,81)	3027 (93,95)
Suburban	30 (3,04)	55 (2,46)	85 (2,64)
Rural	49 (4,96)	61 (2,73)	110 (3,41)

Tooth decay was the most common pathology, averaging 58.7% (1,890 children), followed by dental malposition, 11.3% (968 children).

The prevalence of dental caries in the two provinces was 63.1% in South Kivu and 48.7% in North Kivu respectively. This difference was statistically significant (P<0.05) (Table II).

Table II: Prevalence of dental caries in the provinces of North and South Kivu

Features	Caries prevalence	RP (95% CI)	P-value
North Kivu (n=988)	481 (48,7)	1	
South Kivu (n=2234)	1409 (63,1)	1,18 (1,08-1,28)	<0,001
Total (**n=3222**)	1890 (58,7)		

***PR: Prevalence reports**

A statistically significant difference between dental caries and living environment was noted in South Kivu (p=0.027). In North Kivu, there was no such difference between living environment and the occurrence of dental caries (p>0.05). As for gender, there were no statistically significant associations in either region.

A statistically significant association between dental caries and children's age was found in both provinces, with the risk of caries being higher in children aged 15 (Table III).

Table III: Association between the variables studied and the prevalence of dental caries

Features	Features	% of tooth decay	RP (95% CI)	P-value
North Kivu	Living environment			
	Suburban (n=30)	19 (63,3)	1	
	Rural (n=49)	25 (51,0)	0,60 (0,23-1,52)	0,288
	Urban (n=909)	437 (48,1)	0,53 (0,25-1,13)	0,100
	Total (n=988)	481 (48,7)		
South Kivu	Living environment			
	Suburban (n=55)	25 (45,5)	1	
	Rural (n=60)	30 (50,0)	1,20 (0,57-2,49)	0,627
	Urban (n=2119)	1354 (63,9)	2,19 (1,24-3,63)	0,005
	Total (n=2234)	1409 (63,1)		
North Kivu	Gender			
	Female (n=550)	275 (50,0)	1,06 (0,93-1,21)	0,370
	Male (n=438)	206 (47,0)	1	
	Total (n=988)	481 (48,7)		
South Kivu	Gender			
	Female (n=1220)	790 (64,7)	1,06 (0,99-1,13)	0,071
	Male (n=1014)	619 (61,0)	1	
	Total (n=2234)	1409 (63,1)		
North Kivu	Age (years)			
	5 (n=476)	222 (46,6)	1	
	12 (n=310)	149 (48,1)	1,03 (0,88-1,19)	0,715
	15 (n=202)	110 (54,5)	1,16 (1,09-2,36)	0,035
	Total (n=988)	481 (48,7)		
South Kivu	Age (years)			
	5 (n=1288)	812 (63,0)	1	
	12 (n=434)	250 (57,6)	0,79 (0,83-1,00)	0,045
	15 (n=512)	347 (67,8)	1,27 (1,99-3,15)	0,003
	Total (n=2234)	1409 ,1)		

1.4. DISCUSSION

Tooth decay is a global public health problem that mainly affects the most disadvantaged populations (**52, 53**).

The first study of our work consisted in determining the frequency of dental caries in children in North and Kivu through a retrospective study.

In this study, a caries prevalence of 58.7% was found. These results were similar to those obtained in a study in Canada, where 57% of children aged 6 to 11 had caries, with an average of 2.5 teeth affected (**54**). However, these results are higher than those found by Martens et al. in the dental emergency department of Ghent University, Belgium, in patients aged 0 to 16 (**55**), and those of Tenenbaum et al. who found a prevalence of 42.9% in emergency consultations among children under 16 in the Ile-de-France region (**56**). On the other hand, the prevalence obtained in this study is lower than those of Songo et al. which were 79% and 77.9% respectively in children attending dental clinics and the university clinic in Kinshasa (**57**). The differences observed could be linked to the methods used in the different studies and the age groups considered.

Among the children, 54.9% were female, with a sex ratio of 0.82, which differs from the results found by Songo et al. in Kinshasa (**47**). In our study, 5-year-olds were the most affected (54.75%). This may be due to the fact that at this age children are in nursery school, and most of them consume sugary foods as snacks.

More than half the consultations were carried out on children from urban areas. Geographical access, distance and access time, which raise the issue of health care provision (**10**), could explain these results. On the other hand, a study carried out in Iceland reported that the differences in caries prevalence observed between subjects living in the capital and those living in sites outside the capital were not statistically significant (**58**).

A statistically significant difference in prevalences was noted in both regions. The study by Charles Balagizi et al. in 2018 revealed a high concentration of fluoride in drinking water around the Nyiragongo volcano, which would explain a lower prevalence of dental caries in North than in South Kivu (**59**).

In the present study, the presence of caries was mainly age-related, with the risk of caries being higher in 15-year-olds in both regions.

A statistically significant difference between dental caries and living environment was noted in South Kivu, with a high risk among children living in urban areas. Inadequate dietary practices (snacking, excessive juice consumption) in urban children may explain this susceptibility. These observations are confirmed by Aidara AW and Bourgeois in Senegal, who showed results corroborating the influence of age and living environment on dental caries **(20)**.

Furthermore, a Canadian study showed that the caries rate in children from low-income families was 2.5 times higher than in high-income families **(176)**. According to the same study, much of the burden of dental disease in children was concentrated in disadvantaged groups, namely low-income, aboriginal families.

1.5. CONCLUSION

The results of this first study showed a high prevalence.of dental caries in children aged 5, 12 and 15 attending dental clinics in North and South Kivu.

Study № 2: Prevalence, severity and factors associated with dental caries in children aged 5-6, 12 and 15 years from North and South Kivu.

2.1. INTRODUCTION

Data on the prevalence and severity of dental caries in children and adolescents in North and South Kivu are scarce.

The aim of this study was to assess the prevalence, severity and factors associated with dental caries in North and South Kivu using the ICADS index.

2.2. METHODOLOGY

The survey was a regional, cross-sectional study, running from March to August 2021 among children aged 5-6, 12 and 15 in the 2 capitals (chief towns) of these provinces and in 9 territories.

The study took place in pre-school, primary and secondary schools. The study was carried out according to WHO recommendations for oral health surveys **(61)**, adjusted to the context of the environment. These recommendations suggest three types of community: urban, peri-urban and rural, with 12 sites including 4 sites in the capital, 2 sites in 2 major cities and 4 in rural areas located in different regions **(61).** In this survey, the sites are schools chosen in the capital cities and in various territories of North and South Kivu.

This survey covered pupils aged 5, 12 and 15 enrolled in 20202021. We considered 6-year-olds in elementary school in peri-urban and rural areas, due to the small number of pre-schools where 5-year-olds are enrolled.

This was a cross-sectional survey with three levels of purposive sampling based on accessibility and safety, targeting the capital or the territories on the list of different territories in each province, and students in the selected schools. Certain specific safety, health and accessibility issues led us to make some adjustments to these recommendations.

Since most of the major towns in these two provinces are inaccessible due to the security and health situation (Ebola virus, *etc.)*, the sites were chosen according to the three types of community suggested by the WHO: urban, peri-urban and rural. Thus, 12 schools were chosen in each of the two provinces: 4 urban schools in the capital city (chef-lieu), 4 in peri-urban areas and 4 in rural areas, for a total of 24 schools in the two provinces.

The choice of schools was also based on the consent of the school authorities, enrolment and accessibility. Samples were collected in both public and private schools. Pupils were selected from these schools on the basis of age (5-6, 12 and 15) and parental consent to take part in the study. Characteristics such as absence at the time of the survey or refusal to participate in the study justified non-inclusion in the study.

Data were obtained from the students' interviews and clinical oral-dental examinations.

Variables included: prevalence and severity of dental caries, sociodemographic characteristics, oral hygiene habits (brushing, brushing schedule, frequency and product) and dietary habits (frequency of eating and type of water consumed).

The caries experience was described by assigning ICDAS codes (1-6):

0 = Healthy tooth surface

1 = 1er enamel change

2 = Distinct enamel change

3 = Loss of enamel without visible dentine

4 = Dentine shadow (no dentine cavity)

5 = Distinct cavity with visible dentine

6 = Extended distinct cavity with visible dentine

Severity is defined according to the different ICCMS categories™ (simplification of ICDAS) into healthy faces (ICDAS 0), initial carious lesions (ICDAS 1 and 2), moderate carious lesions (ICDAS 3 and 4), severe carious lesions (ICDAS 5 and 6).

The data collection tool consisted of a pre-tested modified EGOHID clinical questionnaire. Four people, including 2 dentists and 2 students in their final year of public health studies, who had been pre-calibrated and trained, visited the classrooms to carry out an oral examination and collect interview data. The oral examination was carried out under the light of a headlamp, with mirror, OMS probe and 6 probe.

Caries prevalence and severity were calculated using ICDAS criteria.

Quantitative variables were summarized by means and standard deviations. Qualitative variables were presented in the form of frequency and percentage tables. We used Pearson's Chi-square test for comparison of proportions, the

ANOVA test for comparison of variances and *Student's* T-test for comparison of means. A logistic regression model was constructed for variables that were statistically associated with dental caries prevalence in bivariate analyses. *Odds ratios* and their 95% confidence intervals were derived to study the strength of association between variables. The test was considered significant when the p-value was less than 0.05. The number "1" indicated the category with the lowest theoretical risk or with a low proportion.

2.3. RESULTS

The study involved 1,800 children aged 5-6, 12 and 15, with 900 (50%) from North Kivu and 900 (50%) from South Kivu. The sex ratio was 1.06, with 929 (51.6%) boys and 871 (48.4%) girls. According to age and area of residence, the sample was distributed as follows: 600 children (33.33%) were aged 5-6, 600 (33.33%) were aged 12 and 600 (33.33%) were aged 15. Six hundred (33.33%) children lived in urban areas, 600 (33.33%) in peri-urban areas and 600 (33.33%) in rural areas. (Table IV)

Table IV: General characteristics of the sample

Features	N =1800	(%)
Age (years)		
Five-Six	600	33,3
Twelve	600	33,3
Fifteen	600	33,3
Gender		
Female	871	48,4
Male	929	51,6
Zone		
Urban	600	33,3
Suburban	600	33,3
Rural	600	33,3
Province		
North Kivu	900	50,0
South Kivu	900	50,0

The oral health behavior results showed that 79% of students reported brushing their teeth every day. 57% of students said they brushed their teeth once a day, and 50.5% did so in the morning before breakfast. In addition, 67% of students said they used toothpaste and 23% used other products. As for food, 48.11% of students said they ate twice and 36.33% had 3 meals; those who had four or more meals represented 11.11% and 4.44% respectively; as for drinking water, tap water was the most widely consumed (45.28%). 32.33% used spring or river water, 8.5% rainwater and 7.67% lake water. Mineral water was consumed by 5.5% of students, and 0.72% reported consuming the different types of water, as shown in Table V.

Table V: Numbers and frequencies of socio-demographic, oral hygiene and dietary variables

Features	N=1800	(%)
Tooth brushing		
Yes	1420	78,9
No	380	21,1
Brushing frequency /Drs		
Not regular	382	21,2
Once	1019	56,6
Twice	318	17,7
Three times	81	4,5
Brushing schedule		
Morning before meal	909	50,5
Morning and evening after meals	61	3,4
After each meal	82	4,6
No fixed schedule	748	41,6
Brushing products		
Toothpaste	1209	67,2
Other products	415	23,1
No products	176	9,8
Number of meals/day		
2	866	48,1
3	654	36,3
4	200	11,1
More than 4	80	4,4
Type of water consumed		
Tap water	815	45,3
Spring and river water	582	32,3
Rainwater	153	8,5
Lake water	138	7,7
Mineral water	99	5,5

The overall prevalence of dental caries among students in both provinces was 40.89%.

The prevalence of dental caries was higher among children aged 5-6, those living in urban areas and in South Kivu province. This difference was statistically significant ($p<0.05$). On the other hand, there was no difference between gender and the occurrence of dental caries ($p>0.05$).

Table VI: Prevalence of dental caries by gender, age, living environment and province

Features	Prevalence of dental caries/ICDAS
	N= (%)
Gender	**p=0,784**
Female (n= 871)	359 (41,2)
Male (n= 929)	377 (40,5)
Age (years)	**p<0,001**
Five (n=200)	101 (50,5)
Six (n=400)	139 (34,7)
Twelve (n=600)	224 (37,3)
Fifteen (n=600)	272 (45,3)
Living environment	**p<0,001**
Urban (n= 600)	304 (50,6)
Suburban (n= 600)	228 (38,0)
Rural (n= 600)	204 (34,0)
Province	**p<0,001**
North Kivu (n=900)	246 (27,3)
South Kivu (n=900)	490 (54,4)

There was a statistically significant difference between dental caries, brushing frequency and brushing schedule ($p<0.05$). There was also a statistically significant association between brushing product and caries prevalence ($p=0.009$).

The prevalence of dental caries was highest among children eating more than 4 meals. Tap water was more frequently consumed by children. We noted a statically significant association between the type of water consumed and the occurrence of dental caries. This association was not statically significant between the number of meals and dental caries ($p=0.059$).

Table VII: Prevalence of dental caries as a function of oral and dietary hygiene

Features	Prevalence of dental caries/ICDAS
	N (%)
Brushing frequency	**P=0,004**
Not regular (n= 382)	132 (34,5)
Once (n=1019)	419 (41,2)
Twice (n= 318)	142 (44,6)
Three times (n= 81)	43 (53,1)
Brushing schedule	**p=0,002**
Morning before meal (n= 909)	361 (39,7)
Morning and evening after meals (n= 61)	22 (36,1)
After each meal (n=82)	44 (53,6)
No fixed schedule (n=748)	309 (41,3)
Brushing product	**p=0,009**
Toothpaste (n= 1209)	520 (43,1)
Other products (n=415)	160 (38,5)
No product (n=176)	56 (31,8)
Total (n=1800)	736 (40,8)
Number of meals/day	**p=0,059**
2 (n=866)	342 (39,4)
3 (n=654)	262 (40,1)
4 (n=200)	89 (44,5)
More than 4 (n=80)	43 (53,7)
Type of water consumed	**p<0,001**
Tap water (n=815)	407 (49,9)
Spring and river water (n=582)	206 (35,4)
Rainwater (n=153)	39 (25,4)
Lake water (n=138)	43 (31,1)
Mineral water (n=99)	37 (37,3)
Mixed (n=13)	4 (30,7
Total (n=1800)	736 (40,8)

Multivariate logistic regression of socio-demographic characteristics showed that age was not statistically associated with caries prevalence. The risk of caries was also higher in children from South Kivu, with a threefold increase over children from North Kivu.

Children living in urban areas were three times more likely to have dental caries, with a statistically significant difference. (Table VI).

Table VIII: Multiple analysis of socio-demographic characteristics and CAO/ICDAS prevalences

Features	ICDAS prevalence	
	OR aj (95% CI)	P-value
Age (years)		
5-6	1	
12	0,89 (0,70-1,12)	0,343
15	1,27 (0,98-1,56)	0,061
Gender		
Male	1	
Female	1,02 (0,85-1,23)	0,784
Region		
North Kivu	1	
South Kivu	**3,17 (2,60-3,86)**	**0,001**
Zone		
Suburban	1	
Urban	**1,67 (1,33-2,10)**	**0,001**
Rural	0,84 (0,66-1,06)	0,149

Children who didn't brush their teeth were more likely to develop tooth decay, with a statistically significant difference. Both frequency and timing of brushing protected children from tooth decay. The risk of tooth decay according to the ICDAS index was doubled in children who did not use a toothbrush, with a statistically significant association. The risk of tooth decay was multiplied by 2 for children who did not use toothpaste. We also noted that the risk of tooth decay was twice as high in children who drank tap water as in those who drank mineral water, with a statistically significant difference. Children who ate five meals a day had twice the risk of tooth decay, as shown in Table VIII.

Table IX: Multiple analysis of factors associated with prevalences

Features	CAD prevalence		ICDAS prevalence	
	Crude OR (95% CI)	P-value	OR aj (95% CI)	P-value
Tooth brushing				
Yes	1		1	
No	1,31 (0,94-1,83)	0,100	**1,39 (1,09-1,76)**	**0,006**
Daily brushing frequency				
No	0,59 (0,32-1,11)	0,103	**0,46 (0,28-0,75)**	**0,001**
Once	0,65 (0,37-1,16)	0,150	**0,61 (0,39-0,97)**	**0,035**
Twice	1,23 (0,67-2,25)	0,499	0,71 (0,43-1,16)	0,174
Three times	1		1	
Brushing schedule				
After each meal	1		1	
Morning before meal	0,63 (0,35-1,12)	0,119	**0,56 (0,36-0,89)**	**0,013**
Morning after meal	**2,16 (1,01-4,62)**	**0,044**	0,94 (0,53-1,68)	0,857
Evening after dinner	1,18 (0,62-2,24)	0,609	0,43 (0,03-4,95)	0,491
No brushing	0,60 (0,32-1,12)	0,111	**0,45 (0,28-0,73)**	**0,001**
Toothbrush use				
Yes	1		1	
No	1,30 (0,94-1,81)	0,109	**1,38 (1,09-1,75)**	**0,006**
Use of fluoride toothpaste				
Yes	1		**1**	
No	1,30 (0,98-1,72)	0,066	**1,31 (1,07-1,60)**	**0,008**
Use of other brushing products				
Yes	1		1	
No	0,84 (0,61-1,15)	0,295	0,88 (0,70-1,10)	0,270
Type of water consumed				
Mineral	1		1	
Faucet	1,55 (0,84-2,88)	0,153	**1,67 (1,08-2,56)**	**0,018**
Water source or river	1,02 (0,54-1,92)	0,941	0,91 (0,59-1,42)	0,704
Lake	0,99 (0,46-2,13)	0,984	0,75 (0,44-1,30)	0,319
Rain	0,71 (0,32-1,58)	0,412	0,57 (0,33-0,98)	**0,045**
Mixed	1,20 (0,23-6,05)	0,834	0,74 (0,21-2,58)	0,643
Feeding frequency/meal-day				
Two	1		1	
Three	0,80 (0,59-1,07)	0,140	1,02 (0,83-1,26)	0,822
Four	1,29 (0,86-1,92)	0,206	1,22 (0,90-1,67)	0,193
Five	**2,80 (1,70-4,62)**	**0,001**	**1,78 (1,12-2,82)**	**0,013**

The ICCM (simplification of ICDAS scores) classifies caries lesions into three categories according to degree of severity: initial lesions (ICDAS 1 and 2), moderate lesions (ICDAS 3 and 4) and severe lesions (ICDAS 5 and 6).

The distribution of ICDAS scores according to degree of severity showed that 1064 students (59.11%) had an ICDAS score of zero, 456 (25.33%) had initial lesions (ICDAS 1 and 2), 155 (8.61%) had moderate lesions (ICDAS 3 and 4) and 125 (6.94%) had severe lesions (ICDAS 5 and 6).

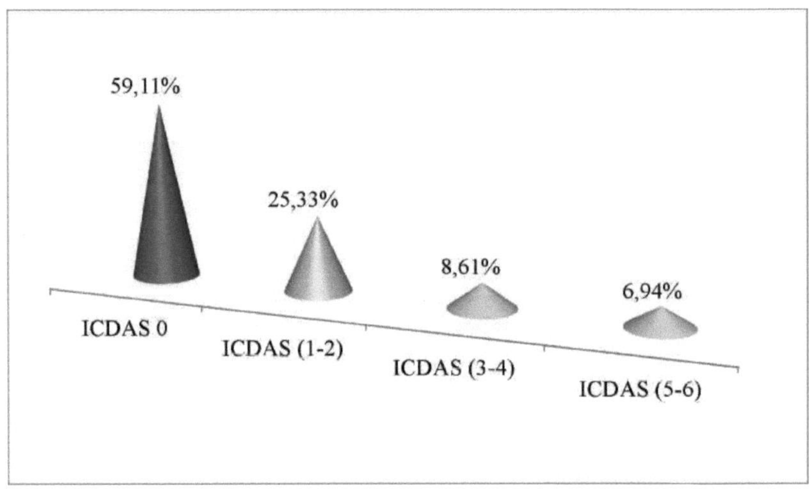

Figure 4: Distribution of ICDAS scores by degree of severity

Our results also showed that children aged 5 years were most affected by dental caries; this association was statistically significant ($p<0.001$). Moderate and severe lesions were more common in boys, while initial lesions were more common in girls, but there was no difference between gender and the occurrence of dental caries ($p=0.5645$).

Depending on living environment and province, dental caries was more prevalent among children in urban areas and in South Kivu, particularly regardless of severity. This association was statistically significant ($p<0.001$).

Table X: Severity of dental caries by age, gender, living environment and province

Features	ICDAS=0 N (%)	ICDAS (1-2) N (%)	ICDAS (3-4) N (%)	ICDAS (5-6) N (%)	P-Value
Age (years)					**P-value<0.001**
Five (200)	99(49,50)	45(22,50)	24(12,00)	32(16,00)	
Six(400)	261(65,25)	76(19,00)	39(9,75)	24(6,00)	
Twelve (600)	376(62,67)	144(24,00)	48(8,00)	32(5,33)	
Fifteen (600)	328(54,67)	191(31,83)	44(7,33)	37(6,17)	
Total (1800)	1064(59,11)	456(25,33)	155(8,61)	125(6,94)	
Gender					**P=0,5645**
Female (871)	512(58,78)	231(26,52)	73 (8,38)	55(6,31)	
Male(929)	552(59,42)	225(24,22)	82(8,83)	70(7,53)	
Total (1800)	1064(59,11)	456(25,33)	155(8,61)	125(6,94)	
Living environment					**P-value<0.001**
Urban	296(49,33)	184(30,67)	61(10,17)	59(9,83)	
Suburban	372(62,00)	149(24,83)	49(8,17)	30(5,00)	
Rural	396(66,00)	123(20,50)	45(7,50)	36(6,00)	
Total(1800)	1064(59,11)	456(25,33)	155(8,61)	125(6,94)	
Province					**P-value<0.001**
North Kivu	654(72,67)	134(14,89)	62(6,89)	50(5,56)	
South Kivu	410(45,56)	322(35,78)	93(10,33)	75(8,33)	
Total (1800)	1064(59,11)	456(25,33)	155(8,61)	125(6,94)	

A statistically significant difference between the severity of tooth decay, brushing frequency and brushing schedule was noted ($p<0.05$). The highest percentage of initial caries was found in students who brushed three times a day after each meal. Moderate lesions were found in those who brushed twice a day but without a fixed schedule. Severe caries was found in those who brushed twice, in the morning and evening, after meals. There were no statistically significant associations with brushing product ($p=0.1046$). Whatever the degree of severity, the highest percentages were found among those who reported using fluoride toothpaste.

Table XI: Severity of dental caries associated with oral hygiene

Features	ICDAS=0 N(%)	ICDAS (1-2) N(%)	ICDAS (3-4) N(%)	ICDAS (5-6) N(%)	P-Value
Brushing frequency					**P<0,001**
Not regular (n= 382)	250(65,45)	83(21,73)	29(7,59)	20(5,24)	
Once (n=1019)	600(58,88)	277(27,18)	86(8,44)	56(5,50)	
Twice (n= 318)	176(55,35)	69(21,70)	32(10,06)	41(12,89)	
Three times (n= 81)	38(46,91)	27(33,33)	8(9,88)	8(9,88)	
Total (n=1800)	1064(59,11)	456 (25,33)	155(8,61)	125(6,94)	
Brushing schedule					**P<0,001**
Morning before meal	548(60,29)	240(26,40)	72(7,92)	49(5,39)	
Morning and evening after meals	39(63,93)	12(19,67)	4(6,56)	6(9,84)	
After each meal	38(46,34)	28(34,15)	8(9, 33)	8(4,56)	
No fixed schedule	439(58,68)	176(23,52)	71(9,49)	62(8,288)	
Total (1800)	1064(59,11)	456 (25,33)	155(8,61)	125(6,94)	
Brushing product					**P=0,1046**
Toothpaste	689(56,99)	319(26,39)	106(8,77)	95(7,86)	
Other products)	263(63,37)	100(24,10)	34(8,19)	18(4,34)	
No products	**112**(63,64)	37(21,02)	15(8,52)	12(6,82)	
Total (n=1800)	1064(59,11)	456 (25,33)	155(8,61)	125(6,94)	

A statistically significant difference was noted between severity of dental caries, frequency of feeding and type of water consumed (p<0.05). Whatever the degree of severity, the highest percentages were found among those who ate four or more meals a day. As for the type of water, the highest percentage of initial and severe caries was found in those who consumed tap water, while moderate caries was found in those who consumed mixed water.

This association was statistically significant (p<0.001).

Table XII: Severity of dental caries associated with food hygiene

Features	ICDAS=0 N(%)	ICDAS (1-2) N(%)	ICDAS (3-4) N(%)	ICDAS (5-6) N(%)	P-Value
Number of meals/day					**p<0,001**
2ndmeal (n=866)	524(60,51)	209(24,13)	72(9,01)	55(6,35)	
3 meals (n=654)	392(59,94)	179(27,37)	48(7,34)	35(5,35)	
4 meals (n=200)	111(55,50)	52(26,00)	18(9,00)	19(9,50)	
More than 4 meals (n=80)	37(46,25)	16(20,00)	11(13,75)	16(20,00)	
Total (n=1800)	1064(59,11)	456(25,33)	155(8,61)	125(6,94)	
Type of water consumed					**p<0,001**
Tap water (n=815)	408(50,06)	253(31,04)	78(9,57)	76(9,33)	
Spring/river water (n=582)	376(64,60)	128(21,99)	49(8,42)	29(4,98)	
Rainwater (n=153)	114(74,51)	24(15,69)	7(4,58)	8(5,23)	
Lake water (n=138)	95(68,84)	25(18,12)	13(9,42)	5(3,62)	
Mineral water (n=99)	62(62,63)	24(24,24)	6(6,06)	7(7,07)	
Mixed (n=13)	9(69,23)	2(15,38)	2(15,38)	0(0,00)	
Total (n=1800)	1064(59,11)	456(25,33)	155(8,61)	125(6,94)	

2.4. DISCUSSION

For the FDI, accessibility to oral health care for the world's poor is a serious problem, and there is an urgent need to raise awareness of the need for preventive oral health care, as well as self-treatment among disadvantaged and at-risk populations. To achieve this, evidence-based models of oral health care need to be developed **(62,63)**. A better understanding of the epidemiological characteristics of oral diseases will enable research to be geared to these needs, and will enable prevention and treatment strategies to be put in place through a combination of individual, community and professional measures. In epidemiological terms, if the prevalence of caries seems to have declined since the end of the 20ème century, this is because the CAD index used by the WHO tends to underestimate the real state of caries, as non-cavitating lesions are not counted (**20**). *The second study* enabled us to assess prevalence, severity using the ICDAS index and factors associated with dental caries in children. To this end, we conducted a study of 1,800 pupils aged 5-6, 12 and 15, enrolled in 24 preschool elementary and secondary schools in North and South Kivu in the DRC. In this study, 51.6% of pupils were male and 48.4% female. These results are similar to those obtained by Leye Benoist et al. among 12-year-olds in Dakar, where boys were the most represented, accounting for 50.41% of cases (**65**). They are contrary to those found in the studies by Aidara and Bourgeois in Senegal **(20)** and Diallo M **(65)** in Mali, where girls were the most represented, accounting for 58.8% and 52.80% of samples respectively. These results also differ from those obtained in a hospital study carried out in the two provinces, where girls predominated (**66).** This difference could be explained by the boy-girl ratio of 5 boys to 4 girls in elementary school in the Democratic Republic of Congo **(66)**, combined, according to the UNICEF 2021 report, with the school attendance deprivation rate among children aged 6-14, which is 27.3% for girls versus 23.9% for boys in North Kivu, and 28.5% for girls versus 26.6% for boys in South Kivu **(67)**.

Of these pupils, 79% said they brushed their teeth every day and 57% did so once a day. Our results are lower than those of Leye Benoist **(64)**, who found that 96% of pupils brushed their teeth daily, including 108 children who brushed twice a day, and those of Diarra.A **(69)**, who found that 93.75% of pupils in his study brushed their teeth. These results could be explained by the non-existence of oral hygiene awareness programs in both provinces. The majority of students ate two meals a day (48.11%). This could be explained by the socio-economic status of the parents. These two provinces are essentially agricultural, with insufficient arable land, agricultural inputs and manpower. Poverty is also very pronounced, with over 80% of the population of North Kivu estimated to survive on less than US$0.20 per person per day (**38**). This situation is at the root of food insufficiency, which results in 36.5% of children aged 4-15 in South Kivu being deprived of proper nutrition (**43**).

As far as drinking water was concerned, tap water was the most widely consumed (45.28%), as it was assumed to be the most potable water supplied by water companies (Régideso, Mercy Corps).

The state of dental health of the subjects in our study is reflected, on the one hand, by the prevalence of caries and, on the other, by the ICDAS index.

The overall prevalence of dental caries among schoolchildren in the two provinces was 40.89%. However, there are relatively few studies using ICDAS in children and adolescents:Aragannal et al, using ICDAS, showed that children and adolescents in India had an average prevalence of 68.8% (**70**). In Spain, a study reported that the prevalence using ICDAS 1-6>0 caries lesions as a threshold for children aged15 years was 84.8%, which is higher than the results of our study Sugar availability and culture-related factors, such as health behaviours, may explain the differences in mean prevalence found between countries (**71**).

In our study, the prevalence of dental caries was higher in 5-year-olds, and 12-year-olds had less dental caries than their 15-year-old peers. These results confirm those obtained in hospital settings in both regions (**66**), where children aged 5 were the most affected (54.75%) and the risk of caries was higher in 15-year-olds. Identical results were reported in Egyptian and Indian children, where the prevalence was higher in temporary than in permanent dentition (**72,73**). This difference may be due to the fact that deciduous teeth are more susceptible to dental caries because of their lower calcium content and structural differences (**74**). Concerning the age at risk, Al-Haj Ali et al (**75**) state that dental health up to early adolescence is likely to be determined by parental knowledge, attitudes and beliefs regarding eating habits and oral hygiene practices, since parents have a leading role and decisive impact on the environment in which children in younger age groups are brought up. By the age of 15, children are in adolescence, a landmark transition period in which family impact gradually diminishes, while openness to influences from the social environment, such as school, peer groups, mass media and youth culture, increases dramatically (**76**). Consequently, behaviors associated with maintaining oral health may be altered during adolescence, such as tooth-brushing practices and eating habits (**77**).

A statistically significant difference between dental caries and living environment was noted, as in the hospital study, with a higher risk in children living in urban areas. The explanatory hypothesis is linked to the process of nutritional transition, which has not yet been completed in peri-urban and rural areas, where the diet is still less industrialized and therefore less cariogenic (**78**). The results of Aidara and Bourgeois in Senegal showed that 42.9% of pupils lived in urban areas and the rest in rural and suburban areas (**20**). Contrary results were found among urban and rural schoolchildren in the Riyadh region of Saudi Arabia (**79**).

We also noted statistically significant differences in the prevalence of dental caries between the two regions, with a higher risk among children in South Kivu. The study by Bahaya MR et al. in 2021 reported a high concentration of protective minerals in drinking water in North Kivu, which would explain a lower prevalence of dental caries in the North than in South Kivu. Similar results have also been found in hospitalized children (**66**).

Tooth brushing plays an important role in preserving oral health: it removes plaque deposited on the surface of the teeth and provides protective fluoride via an age-appropriate fluoride toothpaste (**64**). In this study, however, we found a negative association between tooth decay, brushing frequency and brushing schedule, as children who reported brushing three times a day after each meal and those who reported using toothpaste had a higher prevalence of tooth decay. These results contradict those described in the literature, which show that children who have received oral health education have better dental health. Analysis of the results using multivariate logistic regression, however, showed a high probability and 2-fold increased risk of developing caries in children who didn't brush their teeth and in those who didn't use toothpaste. Brushing schedule was associated with dental caries, as in other studies such as that by Iliana Diamanti in children aged 5, 12 and 15 in Greece (**64,77**).

While oral hygiene has a major influence on the condition of teeth, diet is also an important factor in the fight against tooth decay. Nibbling, and more frequent meals and snacks in general, have been shown to play a part in the caries process (**80**). In this study, we found that children who ate five meals a day were 2 times more likely to develop tooth decay. These results concur with those of a study carried out in Nice on caries risk and schooling zone, which showed that 90.9%

of children consumed sugary foods outside the 3 main meals and a daily snack, and 47% consumed sugary drinks daily outside meals. These children developed more caries than others who were not in this situation (**81**). However, according to Marshall (**82**), a structured eating pattern corresponds to 3 meals (breakfast, lunch and dinner) and 2 snacks, one in the morning and one in the afternoon, representing 5 hours of potential demineralization. When this pattern is unstructured, food intake is more frequent (snacking) and periods of demineralization are longer (**83**). The prevalence of dental caries in many countries has fallen since water fluoridation was first introduced in 1945 (**84**).

Analysis of drinking water in these two provinces revealed that tap water had the lowest fluoride content, while commercial mineral water was almost within the normal range (**85**). This would explain the twofold increase in the risk of tooth decay in children drinking tap water.

The caries data collected reveal that the mean value of ICDAS >0 teeth per child in our study population is 2.11±3.262 for 5-year-olds, 1.2±2.1802 for 6-year-olds, 1.1±2.226 for 12-year-olds and 1.49±2.59 for 15-year-olds. This difference in averages is due to the greater sensitivity of the ICDAS index, to information linked to enamel caries data, and to caries lesions not detectable in CAD surveys being improperly recorded as "*caries free*". The CAD index hides caries that does not require invasive treatment, it hides the total number of caries and their degree of severity, whereas ICDAS shows a greater prevalence of enamel lesions of ICDAS stage 1-2 (reversible caries with prophylactic intervention: remineralization) than of lesions of ICDAS stage 3-4 (where minimal intervention is required) and ICDAS stage 5-6 (needing curative treatment). Similar results were found by Aidara and Bourgeois in Senegal in elementary (age 12) and middle school (age 15) pupils (**20**). Contrary results were obtained by Kouassi (**86**), who showed in a hospital study that the most frequent ICDAS code (>0) was code 5, found in 46.34% of children with temporary dentition.

In the present study, the cross-tabulation of students' caries status with their living environment and province shows that caries involvement for those aged 56 and 12 is significantly related to area of residence (CAO: $p < 0.05$ and ICDAS: $p = 0.001$) and province (CAO and ICDAS: $p < 0.05$). Like the results of MENDES' study of children aged 36-59 months (**87**), those of this study show that gender is not significantly related to caries status. Regarding oral and dietary hygiene, the severity of caries experience was related to brushing schedule and frequency

(ICDAS $p<0.001$). The results of this study revealed a statistically significant relationship ($p<0.05$) for caries severity, feeding frequency and type of water consumed. As with caries prevalence, children who consumed the least fluoridated tap water **(85)** and those who ate more than four meals a day had more severe lesions.

2.5. CONCLUSION

Dental caries remains an irreversible, frequent and unevenly distributed pathology among children aged 5-6, 12 and 15 in North and South Kivu. Analysis of caries according to ICDAS criteria shows a real gain in information, and reveals that the need for prevention (ICDAS 1-2) and interception (ICDAS 34) are higher than the need for curative treatment (ICDAS 5-6).

CONCLUSION AND RECOMMENDATION

The results of this study confirm those of the authors who showed that it was the progression of carious disease towards cavitary lesions (the degree of dentinal damage) that decreased, but not the frequency of carious damage (**88**).

At the end of these studies, we found that dental caries remains an irreversible, frequent and unevenly distributed pathology among children aged 5, 12 and 15 in North and South Kivu. The need for preventive care (ICDAS 1-2) and interception (ICDAS 3-4) is higher than the need for curative treatment (ICDAS 5-6).

The results of this study show poor oral hygiene behavior, with over 50% of children brushing their teeth once in the morning, before eating. More than half of the children reported using fluoride toothpaste, a fluoride supplement that is not available to everyone.

Curative care is rare (treatment index <1): children are less likely to visit health care facilities. This can be explained by difficulties in financial accessibility with impoverished populations; to this must be added an insufficient and unevenly distributed supply of care (18 dentists and 22 structures for the two regions. Preventing tooth decay in children in these two regions (fluoride, food and oral hygiene awareness) remains an effective way of reducing dental caries, while also reducing inequalities in access to oral health care. This prevention must also be taught in schools, starting in kindergarten.

As part of the "Global School Health Initiative", the WHO notes that "schools provide an important setting for health promotion, reaching children, teachers, families and the community as a whole". The school is an essential site for prevention, as it enables early preventive action to be taken, while reducing inequalities in access to health (**29**).

The results of these studies call for this type of survey to be set up in other provinces, in order to harmonize national oral health planning.

REFERENCES

1. Young D.A., Novy B.B., Zeller G.G et al. The American Dental Association Caries Classification System for clinical practice: A report of the American Dental. Association Council on Scientific Affairs. J Am Dent Assoc. 2015; 146: 79-86.
2. Michael G, Orlando MS, Gerhard KS. The FDI Vision 2020: A prospecting of the future of oral health. FDI World Dental Federation.2012; 28p.
3. Marwa M.S. Abbass, Sara Ahmed Mahmoud,Sara El Moshy et al. .The prevalence of dental caries among Egyptian children and adolescences and its association with age, socioeconomic status, dietary habits and other risk factors. A cross-sectional study F1000. Research. 2019, 8:8.
4. Tesfu Z, Duresa A, Mulatu Agajie et al. Dental caries and associated factors in Ethiopia: systematic review and meta-analysis. Envir Health Prev Med. 2021; 26: 21
5. Berkowitz R.J. Mutans Streptococci: acquisition and transmission. Pediat Dent. 2006; 28(2): 106-9.
6. Da Silveira M R. Epidemiology of dental caries in the world. Oral Health Care Pediatric Res Epidemiol Clin Pract. 2012; 8:149-68.
7. Karume K, Bagalwa M, Bagula E et al. Water Quality in and around Lake Edward Basin of the Greater Virunga Landscape, DR Congo Side. J Envir Prot. 2019; 10: 1174-193.
8. Tinanoff N, Baez RJ, Diaz Guillory Cet al. Early childhood caries epidemiology, aetiology, risk assessment, societal burden, management, education, and policy: Global perspective. Int J Paediatr Dent. 2019; 29:238-48.
9. Warren J.J., Van Buren J.M., Levy S.M., et al. Dental caries clusters among adolescents. Community Dent Oral Epidemiol. 2017; 45 (6): 538-44.
10. Programme Nationale de Santé Bucco-Dentaire(RDC). Plan stratégique de la Santé Bucco-Dentaire 2019-2022. 2019; 98p.
11. Wilson Francisco Cruz Rodriguez. Epidemiologia des caries dentales en Republica Democratica del Congo. Fase II Universidad El Bosque Programa de Odontologia - Facultad de Odontologia Bogota DC. 2020; 48p.

12. Ministère provincial du Plan Province du Nord-Kivu (RDC). Localisation des Objectifs de développement durable dans le Nord-Kivu: Rapport provincial. 2017; 152p.

13. United Nations Development Programme. Profil résumé: pauvreté et conditions de vie des ménages, Province du Nord-Kivu; UNDP 2009;20p.

14. Ministry of Health, North Kivu Province. Pyramide sanitaire des zones de Santé. Provincial Health Division. 2020.

15. Ministry of Health, South Kivu Province. Pyramide sanitaire des zones de Santé, Division Provinciale de la Santé. 2020; 66p.

16. Ministère provincial du Plan Province du Nord-Kivu (RDC). Localisation des Objectifs de développement durable dans le Nord-Kivu: Rapport provincial. 2017; 152p.

17. Programme Nationale de Santé Bucco-Dentaire(RDC). Plan stratégique de la Santé Bucco-Dentaire 2019-2022. 2019; 98p.

18. Ana L de Souza, Soraya Coelho Leal, Ewald M Bronkhorst et al. Assessing caries status according to the CASTinstrument and WHO criterion in epidemiological studies. BMC Oral Health . 2014; 14:119.

19. Ana Luiza SC, Maria Isabel PV, Carlos M., et al. Comparison of caries lesion detection methods in epidemiological surveys: CAST, ICDAS and DMF. BMC Oral Health. 2018; 18:122.

20. Aidara A.W, Bourgeois D. Prevalence of dental caries: national pilot study comparing caries severity index (CAO) vs ICDAS in Senegal. Odonto Stomatol Trop 2014; 37(145): 53-63.

21. Braga MM, Oliveira LB, Bonini GA, et al. Feasibility of the International Caries Detection and Assessment System (ICDAS-II) in epidemiological surveys and comparability with standard World Health Organization criteria. Caries Res. 2009; 43(4): 245-9.

22. Ismail AI, Sohn W, Tellez M, et al. The International Caries Detection and Assessment System (ICDAS): an integrated system for measuring dental caries. Community Dent Oral Epidemiol. 2007; 35(3): 170-8.

23. Pitts N. Modern concepts of caries measurement J Dent Res. 2004; 83:43-7

24. Ndiaye A. Epidemiological characteristics and aspects of oral health management in disabled children in Senegal: a study conducted in medico-pedagogical centers. Thesis. Chir Dent. 2009; 22:56p.

25. World Health Organization. Oral health surveys-basic methods. 4th ed.Geneva: WHO; 1997.

26. Pitts NB, Zero DT, Marsh PD et al. Dental caries. Nat Rev Dis Primers. 2017; 3(1): 17-30

27. Marwa MSA, Sara AM, Sara EM et al. The prevalence of dental caries among Egyptian children and adolescents and its association with age, socioeconomic status, dietary habits and other risk factors. A cross-sectional study F1000. Research. 2019; 8:8.

28. Tesfu Z, Duresa A, Mulatu Agajie et al. Dental caries and associated factors in Ethiopia: systematic review and meta-analysis. Envir Health Prev Med. 2021; 26: 21

29. WHO. Regional Strategy for Oral Health 2016-2025, August 19, 2016.

30. Global Burden of Disease. Global, regional, and national incidence, prevalence, and years lived with disability for 354 diseases and injuries for 195 countries and temtories, 19902017: a systematic analysis for the Global Burden of Disease Study. Lancet 2017; 393(10190):44

31. FDI World Dental Federation; The Oral Health Atlas. 2nd Edition. 2015;63p

32. Programme Nationale de Santé Bucco-Dentaire(RDC). Plan stratégique de la Santé Bucco-Dentaire 2019-2022. 2019; 98p.

33. Chabadel O. Caries prevention in children: exploration of individual caries risk and sealing of pits and fissures on temporary molars. Thesis Méd humaine et pathologie. University of Montpellier. 2020; 232p

34. Keyes Ph. Recent advances in dental caries research. Bacteriology. Bacteriological findings and biological implications. Int Dent J. 1962; 12:443-64.

35. FDI World Dental Federation; The Oral Health Atlas. 2nd Edition. 2015;63p

36. Bonner BC, Bourgeois DM, Douglas GV, et al. The feasibility of data collection in dental practices, using codes for the International Caries Detection and Assessment System (ICDAS), to allow European general dental practitioners to monitor dental caries at local, national, and international levels. Prim Dent Care. 2011; 18(2): 83-90.

37. College of Teachers of Pediatric Odontology. Fiches pratiques d'odontologie pédiatrique. Edition CdP. 2014; 347p.

38. Ministère provincial du Plan Province du Nord-Kivu (RDC). Localisation of the Sustainable Development Goals in North Kivu: Provincial report. 2017; 152p

39. Céline la Haye. Drawing Belgian Congo. Ades Dymset. 2006.

40. Ministère provincial du Plan Province du Nord-Kivu (RDC). Localisation des Objectifs de développement durable dans le Nord-Kivu: Rapport provincial. 2017; 152p.

41. United Nations Development Programme. Profil résumé: pauvreté et conditions de vie des ménages, Province du Nord-Kivu; UNDP 2009;20p

42. Kaoutar K, Hilali MK, Loukid M. The situation of dental caries among adolescents in the Wilaya of Marrakech(Morocco). Antropo. 2013; 29:101-8

43. UNICEF. Pauvreté et Privation de l'Enfant en République Démocratique du Congo Rapport Provincial: Province du Nord-Kivu. UNICEF. 2021;8p.

44. USAID From the American People. Monitoring the humanitarian situation - North Kivu Province, DRC .USAID . 2021.

45. Ministry of Health, North Kivu Province. Pyramide sanitaire des zones de Santé. Provincial Health Division. 2020.

46. Ministry of Health, South Kivu Province. Pyramide sanitaire des zones de Santé, Division Provinciale de la Santé. 2020; 66p.

47. Ho L, Labrecque G, Batonon I et al. Effects of a community scorecard on improving the local health system in Eastern Democratic Republic of Congo: qualitative evidence using the most significant change technique. Conflict Health. 2015; 9:27

48. Belhadj L., Metref Z. L., and Serradj S. A., Preliminary dental health survey in children aged 4 to 6 years in Sidi Bel Abbes. J Med Dental Sci Res. 2019; 6 (1): 17-25.

49. Shaghaghian S, Abolvardi M, Akhlaghian M. Factors affecting dental caries of preschool children in Shiraz, 2014. J Dent (Shiraz). 2018;19:100-8.

50. Souza JF, Boldieri T, Diniz MB et al. Traditional and novel methods for occlusal caries detection: performance on primary teeth. Lasers Med Sci. 2013; 28(1): 287-95.

51. World Health Organization. Oral health surveys-basic methods. 4th ed.Geneva: WHO; 1997.

52. Kassebaum NJ, Smith AGC, Bernabé E, et al. Global, Regional, and National Prevalence, Incidence, and Disability-Adjusted Life Years for Oral Conditions for 195 Countries, 1990-2015: A Systematic Analysis for the Global Burden of Diseases, Injuries, and Risk Factors. J Dent Res. 2017; 96 (4): 380-7.

53. Tesfu Z, Duresa A, Mulatu Agajie et al. Dental caries and associated factors in Ethiopia: systematic review and meta-analysis. Envir Health Prev Med. 2021; 26: 21

54. Ronn-Legg A. Children's oral health care-a call to action. Canadian Paediatric Society, Community Paediatrics Committee. Pediatr Child Health 2013;18 (1):44-50

55. Martens LC, Sivaprakash R, Wolfgang J et al. Paediatric dental emergencies: a retrospective study and a proposal for definition and guidelines including pain management. Eur Arch of Paediat Dent. 2018; 19(4): 245-53

56. Tenenbaum. A., Sarric. M., Bas .A et al. Consultations for oral-dental emergencies in children: Retrospective study in Ile-de-France. 2019

57. Songo BF, Declerck D, Vinckier F et al. Caries experience and related factors in 4-6year- olds attending dental clinics in Kinshasa, DR of Congo. Community Dent Health. 2013; 30(4):257-62

58. Agustsdottir H, Gudmundsdottir H, Eggertsson H. et al. Caries prevalence of permanent teeth: a national survey of children in Iceland using ICDAS. Community Dent Oral Epidemiol. 2010; 38 (4): 299-309.

59. Balagizi CM., Kies A, Kasereka M M. et al. Natural hazards in Goma and the surrounding villages, East African Rift System. Springer Science+Business Media B.V., part of Springer Nature. 2018; 93(1):31-66

60. Ronn-Legg A. Children's oral health care-a call to action. Canadian Paediatric Society, Community Paediatrics Committee. Pediatr Child Health 2013;18 (1):44-50

61. Crystal YO, Niederman R. Evidence-based dentistry update on silver diamine fluoride. Dent Clin. 2019; 63(3): 22-9

62. Michael G, Orlando MS, Gerhard KS. The FDI Vision 2020: A prospecting of the future of oral health. FDI World Dental Federation.2012; 28p.

63. Michael G, David MW, Ihsane BY, et al. Optimal oral health for all, vision 2030. FDI .2021; 54p

64. Leye-Benoist F, Bane K, Aidara A et al. Prevalence of dental caries among 12-year-old students in the Dakar region. Odonto Stomato Trop. 2014; (146): 58-64.

65. Diallo I.M. Epidemiology of dental caries in 12-year-old schoolchildren in the commune of Kita through 4 schools. Thèse. Méd. Université Bamako. 2011; N°11: 91p

66. Bahaya MR, Diallo MT, Ndoye S., Prevalence of dental caries among children in Kivu, Democratic Republic of Congo: Retrospective study conducted from 20092019. Rev Col Odonto-Stomatol Afr Chir Maxillo-Fac. 2022; 29(1): 24-29.

67. Programme d'Analyse des Systèmes Éducatifs de la Confem (PASEC); L'enseignement primaire en République Démocratique du Congo; Quels leviers pour l'amélioration du rendement du système éducatif. 2011; 108p.

68. UNICEF. Pauvreté et Privation de l'Enfant en République Démocratique du Congo Rapport Provincial: Province du Nord-Kivu. UNICEF. 2021;8p.

69. Diarra A. Oral status of students at the Institut national des aveugles du Mali (INAM): Chir dentaire, Bamako. 2016; No 288.

70. Arangannal P., Mahadev S.K., Jayaprakash J. Prevalence of dental caries among school children in Chennai, based on ICDAS II. J Clin Diagnostic Res. 2016; 10 (4): 09-12.

71. Kramer AC, Petzold M, Hakeberg M et al. Multiple Socioeconomic Factors and Dental Caries in Swedish Children and Adolescents. Caries Res. 2018; 52: 42-50.

72. Goyal A, Gauba K, Chawla H.S, et al. Epidemiology of dental caries in Chandigarh school children and trends over the last 25 years. J Indian Soc Pedod Prev Dent. 2007; 25(3): 115-18.

73. Marwa M.S. Abbass, Sara Ahmed Mahmoud,Sara El Moshy et al. .The prevalence of dental caries among Egyptian children and adolescences and its association with age, socioeconomic status, dietary habits and other risk factors. A cross-sectional study F1000. Research. 2019, 8:8.

74. Jain A, Jain V, Suri SM, et al. Prevalence of dental caries in male children from 3 to 14 years of age of Bundelkhand region, India. Int J Community Med Public Health. 2016; 3(4): 787-790.

75. Al-Haj Ali S.N and AlShabaab S.H. What do parents know about oral health and care for preschool children in the central region of Saudi Arabia? Pesqui. Bras. Odontopediatria Clin. Integr. 2020; 20:103.

76. West, P. Health inequalities in the early years: Is there equalisation in youth? Soc Sci Med. 1997; 44, 833-58.

77. Iliana D, Elias D.B, Katerina K.,et al. Arapostathis Argy Polychronopoulou ,Constantine J. Oulis. Dental Caries Prevalence and Experience (ICDAS II Criteria) of 5-, 12- and 15- Year-Old Children and Adolescents with an Immigrant Background in Greece, Compared with the Host Population: A Cross-Sectional Study. Int J Envir Res Public Health. 2022; 19: 14.

78. Serigne ND, Sylvie AL, Daouda C et al. Health status, supply and use of oral-dental care among Senegalese children: synthesis of available data. Afrique, santé publique & développement . 2016;28: 257-65.

79. Mohammed A Al-R, Abdullah RA, Ali SA, et al. A Comparison of Dental Caries in Urban and Rural Children of theRiyadh Region of Saudi Arabia. Frontiers Pub Health. 2019;7:195

80. Ho L, Labrecque G, Batonon I et al. Effects of a community scorecard on improving the local health system in Eastern Democratic Republic of Congo: qualitative evidence using the most significant change technique. Conflict Health. 2015; 9:27

81. Muller-Bolla M, Zakarian B, Lupi-Pegurier L et al. Oral health status and individual caries risk according to priority education or non-priority education schooling zone. Epidemiological survey in 2004-2005 in the city of Nice. Rev Odont Stomat. 2006; 35: 219-238.

82. Marshall T.A. Caries prevention in pediatrics: dietary guidelines. Quintessence International. 2004; 35(4): 332-5.

83. Esber Caglar, Ozgur O.Kuscu. The role of diet in caries prevention Springer International Publishing Switzerland. 2016; 196p.

84. Han-Na Kim, Jeong-Hee Kim, Se-Yeon Kim. et al. Associations of Community Water Fluoridation with Caries Prevalence and Oral Health Inequality in Children; International. Journal of Environmental. Res Public Health. 2017;14: 631

85. Bahaya M.R., Bagalwa M., Agbor A.M.,et al. Fluoride and mineral contents in drinking water consumed in South and North-Kivu Provinces, Eastern D.R. Congo. Odonto stomatol Trop. 2021; 44(176): 33-44

86. Kouassi E O. Applicability of L'ICDAS II in temporary dentition: Preliminary study in 41 Senegalese children Thesis: Chir Dent. Dakar. 2014, n°52, 100 p.

87. Mendes FM, Braga MM, Oliveira LB, et al. Discriminant validity of the International Caries Detection and Assessment System (ICDAS) and comparability with World Health Organization criteria in a cross-sectional study. Community Dent Oral Epidemiol. 2010; 38(5): 398-407

88. Agustsdottir H, Gudmundsdottir H, Eggertsson H. et al. Caries prevalence of permanent teeth: a national survey of children in Iceland using ICDAS. Community Dent Oral Epidemiol. 2010; 38 (4): 299-309.

PUBLICATIONS

1. MR Bahaya, Bagalwa Mashimango, Agbor Ashu Michael, Pilipili Muhima Charles, Mushagalusa Nachigera, Karume Katcho, Faye Malick .FLUORIDE AND MINERALS CONTENTS IN DRINKING WATER CONSUMED IN SOUTH AND NORTH PROVINCES, EASTERN D.R. CONGO. Odonto Stomatologie Tropicale. 2021, 44(176): 33-44

2. Bahaya MR ,Diallo MT , Ndoye S , Bagalwa M , Agbor AM , Faye M. Prevalence of dental caries among children in Kivu, Democratic Republic of Congo: Retrospective study conducted from 2009-2019. Rev Col Odonto-Stomatol Afr Chir Maxillo-Fac. 2022; 29,(1):24-29

3. Bahaya MR ,Diallo MT , Ndoye S , Kadimanche M , Faye M. Prevalence of dental caries in children aged 5,12 and 15 years from North and South Kivu in the Democratic Republic of Congo: Etude comparant la Méthode CAO vs ICDAS. Dakar Med. 2022;67(1)

I. IDENTIFICATION AND PERSONAL INFORMATION

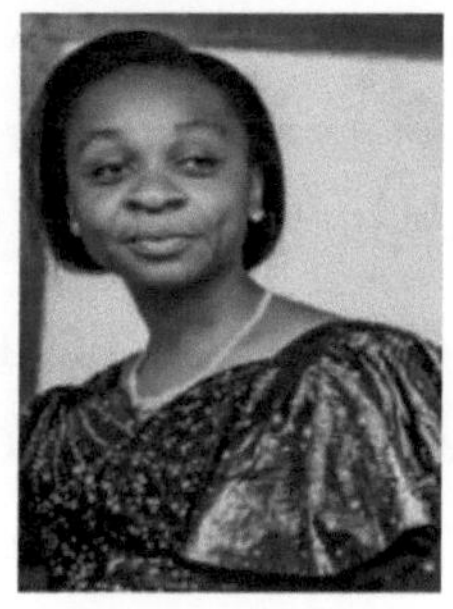

1. APPLICANT'S IDENTITY

Name: BAHAYA MULUZINYERE REINE

Gender: FEMALE

Place of birth: BUKAVU

Date of birth: 07/06/1980

Nationality: CONGOLAISE

Marital status: MARRIED, Mother of 3 children

Dental practice number: 00862

Specialty: PEDIATRIC ODONTOLOGY

2. HOME ADDRESS

Avenue: Corniche No 24 Neighborhood: Muhumba

Commune/territory: IBANDA /Ville de Bukavu/ Province du Sud-Kivu/DR-Congo

3. STUDIES DONE

2018-2022: PhD Thesis/Pediatric Odontology at Cheikh Anta Diop University, Dakar

2015-2018: Master in Pediatric Odontology at Cheikh Anta University Diop from Dakar

2004-2010: Medical studies/dental surgery at Cheikh Anta Diop University, Dakar

2000-2003: Medical studies at the Catholic University of Bukavu/RD-Congo

1992-1999: High school / Biology and Chemistry section at Institut Bwindi

1986-1992: Primary studies at EP KASHUMO/ BAGIRA

4. PREVIOUS JOBS AND EXPERIENCE

- Head of the Department of Dentistry at HGR PANZI
- Member of the Board of Directors of Fondation Panzi/RD-Congo
- Lecturer at the UEA Faculty of Medicine
- Member of the Scientific Committee of the Denis Mukwege International Chair

PUBLICATIONS

1. MR Bahaya, Bagalwa Mashimango, Agbor Ashu Michael, Pilipili Muhima Charles, Mushagalusa Nachigera, Karume Katcho, Faye Malick .FLUORIDE AND MINERALS CONTENTS IN DRINKING WATER CONSUMED IN SOUTH AND NORTH PROVINCES, EASTERN D.R. CONGO. Odonto Stomatologie Tropicale. 2021, 44(176): 33-44
2. Bahaya MR ,Diallo MT , Ndoye S , Bagalwa M , Agbor AM , Faye M. Prevalence of dental caries among children in Kivu, Democratic Republic of Congo: Retrospective study conducted from 2009-2019. Rev Col Odonto-Stomatol Afr Chir Maxillo-Fac. 2022; 29,(1):24-29
3. Bahaya MR ,Diallo MT , Ndoye S , Kadimanche M , Faye M. Prevalence of dental caries in children aged 5,12 and 15 years from North and South Kivu in the Democratic Republic of Congo: Etude comparant la Méthode CAO vs ICDAS. Dakar Med. 2022;67(1)

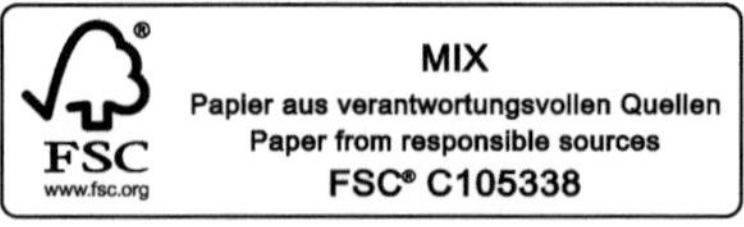

Printed by Books on Demand GmbH, Norderstedt / Germany